MIDDLE SCHOOL

PLUGGED-IN PLANNER

WRITTEN BY

Screen Sanity

IN PARTNERSHIP WITH SUSAN CROWN EXCHANGE

To order additional copies of this resource visit **screensanity.org/tools** or email at **info@screensanity.org.**

HI
THERE.

So glad you're here.

Before you dive in, please take a moment to give yourself a pat on the back — you picked up this planner and are taking action. Kudos to you! Raising kids is not an easy task and the teenage years often feel the most daunting. Add technology into the mix and they're even more intimidating. Our children are facing real risks — cyberbullying, isolation, online predators, comparison, etc. — and it's easy to feel overwhelmed and lost.

We're here to let you know you're not alone. Please remember, there's no perfect way to embark on this journey, and there will certainly be hiccups along the way. As bumpy as the road may seem, it's never too late to take on the challenges of the digital world.

This planner is a guide to help as you step into the ring, preparing for the technology battlegrounds that are already active or on the horizon in your home. Its aim is to help you set intentions, draw boundaries, start conversations and proactively consider the role technology plays in some of your child's formative years.

CONSIDER THE BIG PICTURE

When it comes to device introduction, three words guide our process: **"Ride. Practice. Drive."** Teaching your kid to drive a device is sort of like teaching your kid to drive a car. Similar to driver's ed, there can be an intentional process to introducing new technology.

In navigating this roadmap, it may be helpful to identify where your child is on their digital journey. Take some time to orient yourself on the following map, envisioning what your child's device use will entail in the coming years.

This will look different for every family. The end goal is not to find the magic age or correct plan, but rather to familiarize yourself with the path you plan/hope to take.

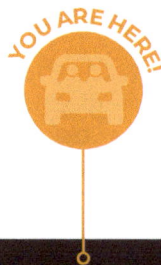

YOU ARE HERE!

| RIDE | PRACTICE | DRIVE |

This planner is focused on supporting parents who are in the passenger seat, helping their kids practice with devices.

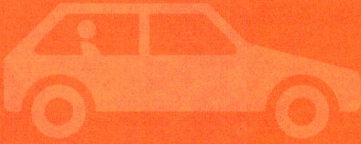

RIDE

Buckle up in the back.

Start by having your child observe your digital practices and device use, similar to how we watched our parents drive from the backseat.

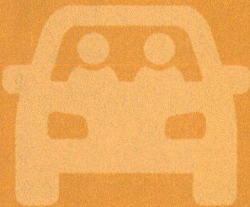

PRACTICE

Start small.

When it's time for a device, consider one that is simple, safe and stripped down to limited features. Allow your kid to experiment with independence and develop foundational skills. During this time, plan to log many hours riding in the passenger seat, helping them practice healthy digital habits.

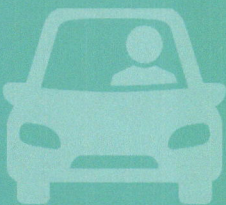

DRIVE

Smartphone independence.

When he or she demonstrates competence and you feel comfortable, your child is likely ready to embark on solo device use. They'll still bump curbs or get into accidents, but they can mostly navigate sticky situations on their own.

1/

THEN
& NOW

It's harder to be a parent than ever before, because it's harder to be a kid than ever before. The core challenges our kids face today are not much different than the ones we grew up with — there are still broken hearts over being cut from the football team or not getting invited to the dance.

Yet, the way we experienced these hardships is quite different from how our kids deal with them today. The digital world allows bullies, comparisons, disappointments and pressures to make themselves at home, right at our kids' fingertips.

Back in the Day

Reflect on your childhood. What experiences are you glad you had before smartphones and social media were introduced? How do these memories help you relate to your child's world?

_____

_____

What pressures do you feel about smartphones or social media in your child's life?

_____

_____

What worries you most about introducing new technology to your child?

_____

_____

⚡ PLUG IN

Growing up Digital

As kids of the '80s and '90s, we could return from school, hang up our coats and leave the outside voices at the door. But for today's digital natives, social media and smartphones leave no room to escape the social sphere. On top of this, **only 14% of youth say they have had a helpful conversation with an adult about their online world.**

One of our most powerful parenting tools is offering connection and empathy to our kids, yet we can't do that without considering what it's like to walk in their shoes. The video below provides a window into what it's like growing up in today's digital age.

Scan to watch the video

2/

START WITH YOURSELF

We recently asked teens to share the number one thing that adults could do to support kids' mental health. Their answer? **"Put down your phones and talk to us."** Ouch.

One of our greatest challenges as modern parents is modeling the digital habits we hope our kids will adopt. Of course, we will never be perfect... but an honest look at our own tech use is a great first step toward building empathy, trust and digital health as a family.

Set aside any pressure to strive for perfect screen habits (here's a secret: they don't exist); rather, give yourself grace and compassion as you reflect honestly on your relationship with screens.

Tech Check

In what ways do your phone and devices add to your life? How do they get in the way?

_____

_____

_____

To support healthy screen habits, you might try **applying friction** — inserting tiny obstacles that make it a little harder to mindlessly reach for your screen. Here are some ideas to get you started:

(1) **Turn off notifications.** Unless they're from real people, it can be freeing to eliminate these tempting little dings that invite us to take "one quick peek."

(2) **Use a watch to filter noise.** Relieve the pressure to have your phone clipped to your hip. A watch can serve as a tool to allow priority people to get through to you, while relieving you from feeling constantly "on call" to the rest.

(3) **Give your phone a spring cleaning.** Give yourself permission to get rid of things that don't spark joy. The app we compulsively open? Try deleting it. That person on Instagram who makes us feel bad about our lives? It's okay to unfollow them.

Other ideas:

○ **Set up charging stations:** Out of sight, out of mind!

○ **Use an alarm clock:** Choose _when_ you want to reconnect in the morning.

○ **Adjust the screentime limits on your device:** Team up with the technology to help you!

Lead with Vulnerability

Share reflections on your own tech habits with your child. If you're feeling particularly brave, you may even add something like, _"I've noticed some-times my tech is actually standing in the way of what matters most. Have you seen this?"_ Inviting this feedback can feel scary, and the answer won't likely be music to your ears — we get it, we're learning from our own kids right alongside you! Listening with curiosity and resisting the urge to defend yourself can open the door to empathetic and honest conversations with your kiddo about screentime struggles.

THINKING ABOUT A PHONE?

Teaching a kid to drive a smartphone is kind of like teaching a kid to drive a car.

You don't hand them the keys and wish them good luck. You start in empty parking lots and on less busy roads before moving to higher traffic areas — offering guided practice to navigate risky situations and road hazards.

When thinking about a phone for your child, take this same "driver's ed" approach. Start simple, with limited options and freedom that grows slowly as your child demonstrates competence, and eventually they will learn to be a self-regulated, independent driver.

Smartphone Roadmap

When deciding on a device, first consider what level of functionality your kid needs. Then, choose a device that meets the need but avoids exposure to more mature experiences. A "first phone", for example, provides basic features that can serve as great training wheels in the pre-smartphone years.

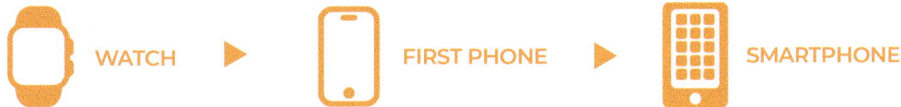

WATCH ▶ FIRST PHONE ▶ SMARTPHONE

What device features do you want your child to have right now? The options you check below can help lead you to the right device.

Text Messaging

- ☐ Family
- ☐ Friends
- ☐ Photo texting
- ☐ Group texting

- ☐ Calling
- ☐ Location tracking
- ☐ Access to educational material
- ☐ Calendar
- ☐ Camera

- ☐ Team communication
- ☐ Entertainment
- ☐ Gaming
- ☐ _____

Looking ahead, what skills do you want your kids to have before they graduate to a smartphone?

- ☐ They turn off/put down their phones without a meltdown
- ☐ They charge their devices outside of their bedroom without reminding
- ☐ They tell me when they update passwords
- ☐ They ask before downloading a new app
- ☐ They come to me when they encounter challenges online and are open to my coaching

Know Your Options

If the responsibility and mental burden of a smartphone isn't the right next step for your family, we want you to know there is a growing market of alternative products. To help in the decision-making process, check out a side-by-side comparison of some of the most popular alternatives on our on our blog.

Scan to visit our blog

INTRODUCING A PHONE

How are we here already?! It seems like just yesterday we were taking off the training wheels and waving goodbye on the first day of kindergarten.

As with many other milestones, the time to enter the world of smartphones sneaks up faster than we may like. How do we prepare our kids (and ourselves) for this rite of passage?

When they've shown they're ready for the responsibility these devices bring, it's helpful to have in mind the boundaries you want to establish. **Start with strong limits and release them slowly,** rather than trying to put them in place during a time of stress.

⊳|◁ **REFLECT**

Unboxing a Phone

Here are some building blocks to consider as you create boundaries for your child's first phone. **Check the ones that feel right for your family.**

☐ **Who owns the phone?**
Giving a phone as a gift can blur the lines of ownership — you might instead present the device as an item on loan (from you, the owner). Your child is still accountable for the decisions made on the device and what happens to it.

☐ **Starting Features**
Phones today come preloaded with a multitude of apps. When setting up your child's phone, it can be helpful to strip it down to its most basic features. For example:

☐ Messaging   ☐ Calculator

☐ Calendar   ☐ Clock

☐ Music Player   ☐ _____

☐ Photo Gallery

☐ **Adding New Apps**
As your child proves successful with the basic features, it's likely they'll soon be asking for more. Here are some tricks to try when your child asks you for an app you don't know much about:

☐ Try it yourself first

☐ Download it on your phone and use it together

☐ Read app reviews (Common Sense Media can be a helpful place to start)

☐ Ask other parents what they know about the app

☐ Ask older youth what they've experienced on the app

☐ **Celebrate the Growth**
Use this moment as an opportunity to tell your child why they have demonstrated they're ready for a phone. Highlight moments your child showed responsibility, trustworthiness and maturity.

⚡ **PLUG IN**

Start the Convo

After reflecting and preparing yourself for this milestone, take time to include your child in the process. Before the plastic wrap comes off and the unboxing begins, share the expectations you've decided upon with your child. Our **Smartphone Toolkit** provides example language for these conversations with your kiddo, as well as fill-in-the-blank worksheet that can be completed together to ensure everyone is on the same page when it comes to the device.

Download the Smartphone Toolkit here

WEAR YOUR SEATBELT

The internet can be like the classic game Nintendo Mario Kart — turtle shells and banana peels flying unexpectedly into view from every direction. Some of these hazards are harmless, yet others can lead to Game Over.

While we'd like to think that these dangers live in the hard-to-reach corners of the internet, the reality is they're only a few clicks away. As your child moves toward device independence, predators, posers, bullies and porn bots have increasing access to your child.

Similar to the ways we prepare our kids for hazards in the physical world, **we can think of these digital precautions like seatbelts, offering as much protection as possible from accidents in the online world.**

Safety First

No solution is 100% foolproof, but applying filters at the router and device level can offer a little peace of mind, minimizing the bumps and bruises your child will encounter in the digital world.

(1) Base Layer. Internet filters at the Wi-fi and router level help keep hardcore content out of your child's Google searches. Take a look at the following options to find the right fit for your family.

- Cleanbrowsing DNS
- Gryphon
- Open DNS
- Circle

(2) Second Layer. Filtering and monitoring at the device level offers protection for when devices leave your Wi-Fi. They scan social media and text feeds, alerting you when there is harmful content. We've found the following options to be trustworthy and worthwhile:

- Bark
- Canopy
- Covenant Eyes

(3) Safety Nets. Because we love our kids, we don't want to send them into the digital world unprotected. Here are some best practices to help your family avoid the hazards of the digital world.

- Set expectations about where the device is used (avoid allowing use in private, like bedrooms and bathrooms)
- Turn off location on device
- Block messages/calls from strangers
- Keep passwords shared and up to date

Poker Face

Even with safety nets in place, mistakes happen. When your child shares — or you uncover — an awkward or shocking situation, it's critical you don't overreact. Make it clear to your child that nothing they could ever do or see online will change the way you love them. Pick a phrase you want to practice to help you keep your "poker face."

- Tell me more.
- Thanks so much for trusting me with this.
- Gosh, that's hard. How did that make you feel?
- I'd love to hear more. Want to grab some ice cream?
- I'm so glad you know you can tell me anything.

BABY STEPS TO SOCIAL MEDIA

As our kids age, they're met with a set of "unspoken rules" they begin to internalize. Girls should be tall, but not too tall. Boys fit, but not too muscular. Don't mess up, or you face the risk of cancel culture.

These messages appear from many angles — books, TV shows, movies, etc. — and are especially prominent in the scrolling feeds of social media. We encounter these same "rules" as adults, yet our pre-frontal cortexes are fully developed to step in with higher reasoning and critical thinking.

We're able to decipher what's true from what isn't. As our kids get ready to enter this arena, it's important we show them how to do the same.

▷|◁ **REFLECT**

The Learner's Permit

When thinking about social media for your child, adopt the same "driver's ed" mentality. Prepare your child with small, supported steps before they dive in fully. Here are a few ideas for a social media "learner's permit".

Supervised Practice

☐ **Start with a family account**
This can be a great way to dip toes into social media, sharing pictures of your family pet or your cooking adventures in the kitchen.

☐ **Tour your social media**
Show your child examples of accounts you do and don't like, offering context to why you feel that way. Share your observations and feelings about topics such as body image, violent or graphic content, FOMO, comparison, unrealistic standards, filtered images, etc.

☐ **Begin on your phone**
When it's time for them to try their own account, start on your device, where you can approve all the posts initially and only allow a limited number of friends or family.

Coach Through the Hazards

☐ **Explain the traps**
Prepare your kiddo for the different techniques social platforms use to keep us hooked on our feeds, explaining that these sites are designed to capture their attention through curated content. It may be helpful to watch the Netflix documentary *The Social Dilemma* to start the conversation.

☐ **Show your child how to block and report inappropriate content**
Help them identify where the potholes and fender benders are likely to occur on the app and make an exit plan.

☐ **Model critical thinking**
Help your child be a critical consumer of the information that's bound to flood their feeds. Start with something small or trivial — pointing out that the Big Mac in an ad looks quite different than what comes through the drive-through window — to bridge into more complex examples.

⚡ **PLUG IN**

Social Media Playbook

As a prerequisite, before your kid gets any social media accounts, check out our highly recommended **Social Media Playbook.** It will help you establish clear expectations, norms, and open lines of communication with your kids. Social media is one of the scariest places in the online world, leaving pitfalls for our kids around every corner. This workbook is incredibly helpful in prepping your child for navigating the hazards of social media.

7 /

TIME TO RECHARGE

Our devices can be beautiful tools for productivity and connection — however, if you picked up this book you know the world of screens is not so straightforward.

These incredible devices can be quiet thieves of our attention and sleep. **80% of teens report checking their phones throughout the night, often responding to every notification.**

Like setting a curfew, creating a device bedtime can remove some pressure from our kids.

▷|◁ REFLECT

Setting Structure

What are times and spaces where you hope to create device-free zones? Don't feel like you need to do them all — just choose 2-3 that are right for your child.

- ☐ Bedrooms
- ☐ Bathrooms
- ☐ During meals (even if they're drive-through on the way to practice!)
- ☐ Vacation
- ☐ In the car (except long trips)

- ☐ Before school
- ☐ During school
- ☐ Sports practices/games
- ☐ When friends are over
- ☐ During homework
- ☐ _____

Thinking about establishing a device bedtime? Start by finding a good spot in your home for devices to recharge at night. Here are some ideas:

- ☐ Kitchen
- ☐ Parents' room

- ☐ Home office
- ☐ _____

⚡ PLUG IN

Healthier Coping Habits

If a device has already found a home in your child's room, it may be jarring to abruptly remove it completely. Our kids can become dependent on their devices for emotional regulation. When setting a device bedtime you may want to take the following two steps:

1. **Uncover any reasons for resistance.** Have a conversation with your child, listening to the "why" behind their desire for the device. Worries or fears about fitting in? Stress surrounding social drama or keeping up with social media? Escapism through gaming, mindless scrolling, video viewing? Carrying the burdens of other teens?

2. **Talk with other parents.** One of the most difficult parts of setting a device bedtime is the FOMO that settles in. The idea that "everyone else is doing it," has a powerful hold on our kids. Talk with the parents of your kid's friends to see if the entire friend group can agree to a device curfew.

Scan the QR code to read more about one family's experience implementing a device bedtime in our viral blog post ***Our Daughter's Nightly Struggle.***

CREATE +
CONNECT >
CONSUME

Screentime can drain our mental health, but if we're intentional, technology can also be used as a tool to support it. Instead of being platforms of consumption, **screens can be used purposefully to spark creation.**

One of the most forward-thinking things we can do as parents is team up with technology, helping our kids see it as a means to an end — a mode for driving creativity, curiosity and connection — and not the goal itself.

Plugged in with a Purpose

We often divide our interactions with technology into three categories: creation, consumption and connection. What are some ways your child's screen use falls into each of the following? Here are a few ideas:

Creation	Connection	Consumption
☐ Finding new recipes	☐ Video calls with family members	☐ Watching movies/ videos
☐ Designing graphics	☐ Messaging friends	☐ Scrolling social media
☐ Creating PowerPoint presentations	☐ Watching a show with others	☐ Listening to music or podcasts
☐ _____	☐ _____	☐ _____

It can also be rewarding to have your child use their devices in ways that prepare them for when they leave our homes. We love these ideas for building independence and foundational skills.

☐ Ordering takeout online or over the phone

☐ Scheduling haircut, dentist or doctor's appointments

☐ Entering the address and planning the navigation route

☐ Drafting an email to a family member

☐ Conducting basic internet research for you

☐ Making PowerPoint presentations for fun

☐ Designing the birthday party invite

These helpful tips come from Melissa Griffin (aka "HR Mom"), an influencer and HR executive who has developed internship programs at companies like Petco and Nationwide.

⚡ PLUG IN

Connect with Creativity

Take some time to reflect on how you connect with your creative side and see if you can exercise that muscle in your digital world. Start small in one area — say, social media. Can you replace some of your scrolling with intentional research, discovering more about something you're passionate about? Can your posts become an outlet for creative writing? Once you experiment with this concept, invite your kiddo to join you in engaging with technology in a higher quality way.

FIND YOUR VILLAGE

Raising kids in this digital world is hard, but it's even harder to do it alone. One of the best ways you can stay in the game is finding other parents and influential voices to link arms with when it comes to screentime.

It can be overwhelming to start a conversation about screentime with others — but the sooner you start, the more you will benefit and "get ahead" of the challenges to come.

Technology is the number one battleground in homes today and by taking the time to connect with others in your circle, you'll likely realize they're struggling with it, too!

Roll Call

Who are the parents of your child's closest friends? How do you feel they approach technology and would you feel comfortable talking to them?

_____

_____

Is there someone you feel safe talking to — maybe even one of the names above — as you navigate the challenges of raising kids in a digital world?

_____

_____

Is there someone who you need to communicate with regarding screentime boundaries or concerns? (eg., grandparents, friends' parents) What are your hesitations — and what is the best possible outcome?

_____

_____

⚡ PLUG IN

Stand Together

As parents, we share everything from carpool duties to tutor recommendations to game-day snacks. When it comes to screentime, starting a Screen Sanity Group Study or hosting a Screen Sanity Parent Night can be great ways to create a safe, non-judgmental space to answer the questions we're all pondering.

Visit **screensanity.org** for more information about bringing Screen Sanity to your community, school or group.

You were never meant to do life alone, so let's continue this journey together!

Screen Sanity is here for you at each milestone and tech-related challenge.

Continue to stay connected with our companion workbook,
the Social Media Playbook and our hallmark product, the Screen Sanity Group Study.

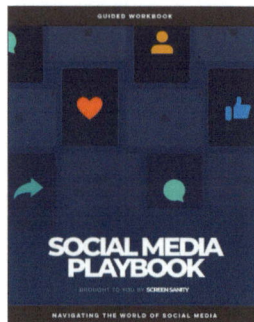

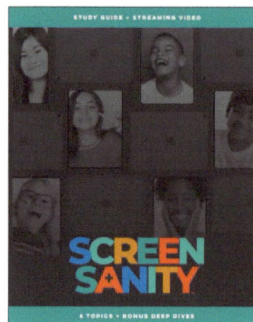

SCREENSANITY.ORG

Notes

www.ingramcontent.com/pod-product-compliance
Lightning Source LLC
Chambersburg PA
CBHW041106050426
42335CB00047B/172